Escape
Nightmares

A WTL SHORT BOOK

Escape Nightmares

Copyright © 2018 WTL International

Published by
WTL International
930 North Park Drive
P.O. Box 33049
Brampton, Ontario
L6S 6A7 Canada

www.wtlipublishing.com

ISBN 978-1-927865-30-9

Printed in the USA and Canada

10 9 8 7 6 5 4 3 2 1

ESCAPE
NIGHTMARES

By Rev. Dr. Moses G. Agyei "Dream Doctor"
and Aisha D. Hammah

TABLE OF CONTENTS

INTRODUCTION

There are different forms of dreams that can affect people's lives in every sphere either positively or negatively. The most troubling one among them is the nightmare. Those who have frequent nightmares may find their minds, souls, spirits and bodies get affected. It is not just one's sleep-life that is touched. As a result, some take their lives or cause self-harm if not dealt with early enough. Sometimes, everyone around the victim gets affected as well. The worse thing to do is give up on yourself or others experiencing this. In fact, it is heartbreaking to see one's spouse, child, sibling or other loved one going through the turbulence of frequent nightmares, especially when all medical attempts prove futile but there are some things that seem to work. It is for this reason this book was made. We seek to guide families, friends and the victims to deal with nightmares since everyone is vulnerable to this horrible form of dream.

WHAT ARE NIGHTMARES?

A nightmare is an unpleasant dream. Nightmares often cause fear but also can trigger feelings of despair, anxiety and great sadness. Nightmares are usually more vivid than most normal dreams. Some nightmares make your "skin crawl" and some are like torture.

Nightmares leave you feeling upset, tired, deserted, scared and powerless. Some people experience nightmares frequently and some only occasionally, but anyone who has had one knows that even one nightmare can be traumatic. It's easy to become a slave to nightmares so it's important to know how to rid yourself of them.

One sleep-time phenomenon that can be classified as a nightmare experience is sleep paralysis. Have you ever been half-awake—half-asleep and felt like you couldn't move your body and/or like something was on top of your chest? That's sleep paralysis. It often comes with mild to intense hallucinations, sensory perceptions and vivid, unpleasant dreaming. This age-old torturous phenomenon is experienced frequently by a large portion of the population.

WHERE WE'RE COMING FROM

We have gathered a lot of experience with dreams over the years and we happen to embrace a Christian perspective, but we hope you'll find this Christian perspective on dreams helpful even if you're not a Christian.

Based on assessing hundreds and hundreds of clients and thousands of dreams over the years, we have identified some common threads that connect waking behaviors and nightmare patterns.

No offense is intended to those who hold dear some of these behaviors we will warn about. We're trying to be helpful, tell what we have come to believe is the truth, and report what we've found to help you escape your nightmares.

Some Dreams are Spiritual

Due to today's culture and because we often get very busy with our lives on the surface, we often forget there is a spiritual aspect to the world and the dreams we have. Ironically, there's actually a lot more going on in the spiritual realm than the physical. We can look at the physical as just a small reflection of the spiritual.

Dreams are often spiritual in nature and may give birth to physical realities that either harm us or do us good. Ever wonder how a dream can express a thought or idea that you don't come up with yourself? Such dreams show that intelligent ideas can originate outside of our own minds. Any other form of intelligence that originates outside of us can be classified as coming from one's encounter with the Spirit of God or the realm of the soul or the spirit. Our biochemistry alone is not capable of forming such thoughts. Thus we can conclude there are spiritual being(s) in the unseen realm capable of forming intelligible ideas and downloading them in our souls or spirits.

SOME NON-SPIRITUAL SOURCES OF NIGHTMARES

Traumatic events. Events that are particularly traumatic can leave you with terror. It could be abuse, an accident, a natural disaster or death. The terror that results hijacks your mind and when you sleep, you experience dreams related to the trauma.

Mental illness. A mental disorder can trigger bad dreams. A lack of counsel or a disorganized life can create extra tension in your mind that leads to nightmares.

Emotional issues. Experiences like marriage crises, divorce or seeing a loved one suffer can send us on a reel of extreme emotions. This creates a breeding ground for nightmares.

Poor self-care. Not taking good care of yourself can result in nightmares. For instance, if you don't take care to get enough rest, fatigue can send your thoughts awry—including your "nightly thoughts." Similarly, if you don't get proper nutrition, an imbalance could leave you in a highly irritable mood and the negativity can magnify/shift your emotions, which in turn can trigger nightmares.

Most of These sources May Be Ultimately Spiritual

We argue that ultimately, most of these sources of nightmares may be spiritual. Many times, if you go back far enough, you will be able to arrive at a spiritual cause. Consider someone who is having nightmares because he doesn't take proper care of himself. Imagine we discover the person is not eating well because he has some degree of a mental imbalance. The mental imbalance was set off at the time of an emotional upset. The upset was set off because he was spiritually compromised. At the end of the day, it was spiritual, and this is what we sometimes find.

SOURCES OF SPIRITUAL NIGHTMARES

At the spiritual level, nightmares come from two main sources: a nightmare can be Godly or it can come from Satan. Dreams are God's and Satan's territory. We have nothing to do with making them. Can you make yourself or someone else dream? This indicates that dreams are beyond human capabilities. *From God*, you ask? This is not a new belief. In the book of Job from the Bible, the godly man Job describes being terrified by "visions of the night" as a way God helped him deal with pride (Job 4:12-17; 33:14 -18). From the dream of Job, we might deduce that a nightmare may be sent by God to help you or to warn you where any other dream would be taken less seriously.

Most of the time, a nightmare is related to Satan and his agents. Satan exists and he may be trying to make you fearful; disbelieve God exists; accept that bad things just happen in life and you can't do anything about them; or make you feel God can't really help.

SOURCES OF SPIRITUAL NIGHTMARES, CONTINUED

In some parts of the world, it's common to believe that someone may actually be deliberately dabbling in the spiritual realm using satanic powers against you. Such activity could expose you to nightmares as a side effect. It is not a new idea that without a spiritual defense, you can fall victim to nightmares from satanic sources.

Interestingly, we believe most often, nightmares come from innocent exposure to sin, spiritual pacts and principles, demonic activity and even demonic objects. Satan tries his best to expose everyone to these.

Nightmares are almost always related to your exposure to one of these spiritual channels. And because God has given every person the power to overcome evil and a knowledge of what to avoid, this can become either your fault or your victory.

CHANNELS OF SPIRITUAL EXPOSURE: THE BAD ONES

There are some obvious channels and some less obvious channels that most of us fall under at some point in time and we must free ourselves from them. It shouldn't surprise you that many people experience nightmares after engaging in the things we've all heard that the God of Abraham, Isaac and Jacob prohibits. Most of us know these are "bad" to do. Idolatry, witchcraft, satanic worship and bestiality are some of them (1 Corinthians 6:9-12; Revelation 21:8; James 4:7; Exodus 22:19). These are channels that expose you to nightmares that are rather easy to avoid if your heart is set to please God.

CHANNELS OF SPIRITUAL EXPOSURE: THE "OKAY" ONES

Then there are a number of channels that you know are prohibited by the God of Abraham, Isaac and Jacob, but you think of them as harmless or "okay." Many of us find ourselves doing them. These are activities like visiting medicine men or people who consult the dead. Depending on where you live, those activities may seem foreign, but instead of a chicken sacrifice filled with blood in a dark hut somewhere, think of seeing the psychic palm reader at the mall, consulting the daily horoscope in the paper or the wooden idol god you put in your garden. These count too. As you stretch your imagination, you can appreciate how such channels seep into the everyday lives in every culture around the world.

CHANNELS OF SPIRITUAL EXPOSURE: THE TRICKY ONES

Some channels of exposure to nightmares are even more innocent-seeming. These consist of things like some games and festivities, some cultural ordinances, the reading of strange books, praying to Mother Nature, or hanging onto demonic trinkets you keep but you may not even know that someone has devoted it to some god. Even idolatry can seem innocent at times. You bring home a figurine which is supposed to bring good luck or a "frog prince" statue and you give it a kiss on the cheek like in the frog prince story. You halfheartedly believe it may bring a husband into your life. The frog has no power to bring you the right person; only God does. Anything you spend more time on than your relationship with God, you break one of God's rules for, or you replace with God is an idol. It can be tricky, but if you can recognize these channels for what they are, they're pretty obvious too.

Channels of Spiritual Exposure: The Hidden Ones

Rites and pacts made by ancestors. It is believed that rites, oaths and covenants (or pacts) our forefathers made expose us to the spirit world. We don't know much about this or how it works, but rites and pacts were a big part of society in the past though the God of Abraham, Isaac and Jacob forbade them. They weren't just empty actions but had spiritual implications (Lamentations 5:7).

Curses. A curse is a spiritual transaction that results in ill fate. The resulting ill fate may be in one area of a person's life, like nightmares, or multiple areas. It's difficult in our very physical society to think of spirits, demons and curses. But these can be very real. It is possible a series of nightmares may result from a spiritual transaction made that involved you.

CHANNELS OF SPIRITUAL EXPOSURE: THE BIG ONE

Masturbation. There's just something that isn't quite right about masturbation. We go about our lives and the way we go about sex seems habitual to us, but activities like masturbating, getting aroused to strange or forbidden themes and other things you might have come to find normal in your personal life may expose you to demonic attacks and nightmares. We find that sleep paralysis in particular is very often tied to illicit sexual behavior, especially masturbation. This has been a secret of Satan's. Some doctors and scientists say that masturbation is normal and even a must, but this is not scientifically proven. On the contrary, something seems to link masturbation with abnormal sleep patterns, nightmares and sleep paralysis. This type of self-serving sexual activity seems to open up one's soul to demonic activity and nightmares consistently unlike any other channel today. It's good news because there is something you can do about it.

YOUR DAILY DEFENSE

We cannot change experiences like past traumatic events, mental illness and incidents that trigger emotional issues. Even managing poor self-care that may be a sign of a deeper problem may be difficult, but we can change our spiritual life. Fortunately, how we govern our spiritual life and interact with God may bring better outcomes with the non-spiritual sources of nightmares, while it may also steer us clear of the channels for spiritual exposure to nightmares. It has been proven that a healthy spiritual life can help a person to overcome past traumatic events, mental illness, emotional issues and poor self-care. Thus, attacking nightmares by addressing our spiritual lives can be most effective. Here is what you can do.

WHAT YOU CAN DO

1 Stop these activities and get rid of all objects of the occult. Spiritual experts usually recommend going as far as burning them not just throwing them away (Acts 19:18-19). Stopping masturbation may be the toughest. It takes identifying what leads you down that path and having zero tolerance for these triggers that lead to the full deed.

2 Test it out. Avoid these channels we suggest expose you to nightmares and see if the frequency of nightmares subsides.

3 Release yourself from past exposures with a prayer. For an optimal life, everyone at some point needs to consciously draw upon the power of God to be fully released from past exposures by officially denouncing them. It might seem a little silly, but try praying something like this: "God, if you're listening, please forgive me of all my sins, wash my spirit clean and deliver me from the power of nightmares and any past rites, pacts, curses, etc. I denounce my involvement in any occult activities. Amen."

WHAT YOU CAN DO, CONTINUED

4 Study and analyse your nightmare experiences. God may use nightmares to prompt you to action concerning satanic agendas. He may want you to pray or take other actions to avert them. Sounds a little weird, but there may be clues in your dreams. Sometimes godly nightmares persist because we never study what God may be trying to say to us.

5 Consider building a genuine relationship with Jesus Christ. Jesus has been said to be the one and only solution against all negative spiritual powers and curses whether demonic, satanic, Adamic, ancestral, generational or other. It is said that God has provided the solution through His death and resurrection. And since God can do anything, knowing Him more, obeying and consulting Him is a good solution for both sources of nightmares. When you know Him, it's not a matter of remembering a long list of things you can't do. You have a Father who can guide your heart and point out specific traps to avoid.

What You Can Do, Continued

6 Try using the name of Jesus. Philippians 2:9-11 says that His name is above every name and at that name, all spirits must bow. Some people have mastered consciously saying "Jesus" during their nightmare experiences, even as actors in their dreams, and they believe this helps make them go away. It can't hurt trying to call on Jesus' name at night.

7 Whenever it looks grim, try to embrace a positive attitude, believing that nothing can take control of your life and enslave you, not even nightmares. Sometimes doing the opposite, thinking the nightmares are in control of your life, shows that you believe that nightmares are bigger than God. Your outlook is a key factor. Don't give the power to nightmares with an attitude of defeat. You have the potential to take back the power.

Remember...

Remember, nightmares often serve as flags that something is wrong in a spiritual area of your life. Although we are victims of nightmares in a sense, we are victims only because we fall into traps enabled by our own sin. The power for a better outcome is in your hands. You are in charge of your spiritual life. Once you know this, the only thing that can keep you enslaved by nightmares is yourself by neglecting to do the work, addressing it biblically. Who knows why God allows nightmares? They're pretty scary and worrisome. However, one thing we know is that they may cause you to sort out your spiritual life for the better, and in the process, they call you to become a better you, spiritually, and by extension, physically, emotionally and mentally.

THE END

www.ingramcontent.com/pod-product-compliance
Lightning Source LLC
Chambersburg PA
CBHW080058280326
41934CB00014B/3360